Thyroid Cookbook

MAIN COURSE – 60+ Breakfast, Lunch, Dinner and Dessert Recipes to heal Hypothyroidism and restore thyroid health

TABLE OF CONTENTS

Introduction

Thyroid recipes for personal enjoyment but also for family enjoyment. You will love them for sure for how easy it is to prepare them.

TOASTED OATMEAL WITH SPICES

Serves: 2
Prep Time: 5   Minutes

Cook Time: *10*   Minutes

Total Time: *15*   Minutes

INGREDIENTS

- 1 cup gluten- free oats
- 2 cup water
- 1 cup unsweetened coconut
- 1 tsp vanilla extract
- ¼ tsp cinnamon
- ¼ tsp nutmeg
- 1 tablespoon coconut oil
- 1 apple
- 1 tablespoon maple syrup

DIRECTIONS

1. In a saucepan heat coconut oil, add oats and coconut flakes and toast for 2-3 minutes

2. Add water, milk, vanilla, nutmeg and stir

3. Serve with apple slices, cinnamon and maple syrup

Serves: *2*

Prep Time: **5**   Minutes

Cook Time: ***15***   Minutes

Total Time: ***20***   Minutes

INGREDIENTS

- 2 cups unsweetened coconut milk
- 1 tablespoon maple syrup
- 1 tsp turmeric
- 1 tsp cinnamon
- 1 tsp gingerroot

DIRECTIONS

1. In a saucepan add all ingredients, except cinnamon
2. Bring to a boil and simmer for 5-10 minutes
3. When ready remove from saucepan and serve with cinnamon

Serves: *8*

Prep Time: *10* Minutes

Cook Time: *10* Minutes

Total Time: *20* Minutes

INGREDIENTS

- 2 medjool dates
- ¼ cup butter
- ¼ cup desiccated coconut
- ¼ cup walnuts
- 2 tablespoons banana flour
- Stevia extract
- ¼ tsp cinnamon

DIRECTIONS

1. In a blender add all ingredients and blend until smooth
2. Remove from the blender and roll into balls
3. Sprinkle with coconut and refrigerate
4. When ready remove from the fridge and serve

Serves: *1*
Prep Time: **5**   Minutes

Cook Time: **5**   Minutes

Total Time: ***10***   Minutes

INGREDIENTS

- 1 tsp basil leaf
- ¼ tsp lemongrass
- ¼ tsp cinnamon pieces
- 1 tsp honey
- 1 lemon wedge

DIRECTIONS

1. In a teapot add basil, cinnamon and lemongrass
2. Add boiling water and let it chill for 4-5 minutes
3. Remove the tea bag, add honey and serve

Serves: **1**

Prep Time: **5** Minutes

Cook Time: **5** Minutes

Total Time: **10** Minutes

INGREDIENTS

- 1 cup water
- ¼ cup hemp seeds
- 1/4 beet
- 1 tablespoon ghee
- 1 tsp honey
- 1 tsp vanilla extract

DIRECTIONS

1. **In a blender add all ingredients and blend until smooth**
2. **Pour into a cup and serve**

Serves: *1*

Prep Time: *10*   Minutes

Cook Time: *15*   Minutes

Total Time: *25*   Minutes

INGREDIENTS

- 1 cup water
- ¼ cup pecans
- 1 tablespoon honey
- 1 tsp vanilla extract
- ¼ tsp nutmeg
- ¼ tsp cinnamon
- ¼ tsp cloves
- salt

DIRECTIONS

1. In a blender add all ingredients and blend until smooth
2. Pour into a cup and serve

Serves: **8-10**

Prep Time: **10** Minutes

Cook Time: **50** Minutes

Total Time: **60** Minutes

INGREDIENTS

- 2 beets
- 1 avocado
- ¼ cup blueberries
- ¼ cup raspberries
- 1 tsp vanilla extract
- 2 tablespoons maple syrup
- 1 cup cacao powder

DIRECTIONS

1. In a saucepan bring water to a boil
2. Add beets and cook until tender
3. Blend the beets with avocado, raspberries, blueberries and maple syrup
4. Add cacao powder mix well and refrigerate for 1-2 hours

5.   Spoon out mixture and roll into balls and serve

15

Serves: *4*
Prep Time: *10*   Minutes

Cook Time: *10*   Minutes

Total Time: *20*   Minutes

INGREDIENTS

- 2 tablespoons maple syrup
- 1 cup coconut milk
- 1 tablespoon lime zest
- ¼ cup lime juice
- 1 tsp vanilla extract
- 1 tsp salt

DIRECTIONS

1. In a saucepan add all ingredients and bring to a simmer
2. Whisk until pudding thickens
3. Pour into ramekins and serve

Serves: **2**

Prep Time: **10** Minutes

Cook Time: **10** Minutes

Total Time: **20** Minutes

INGREDIENTS

- **2 cups tart cherries**
- **1 banana**
- **¼ tsp ground star anise**

DIRECTIONS

1. **In a blender add all ingredients and blend until smooth**
2. **Pour mixture into ramekins and sprinkle coconut flakes**
3. **Serve when ready**

Serves: *8*

Prep Time: *10*   Minutes

Cook Time: *30*   Minutes

Total Time: *40*   Minutes

INGREDIENTS

- 8 apples
- 1 cup poppy seeds
- ¼ cup honey
- 1 tablespoon vanilla extract
- 1 cup pecans
- ¼ tsp all spice
- 1 tablespoon honey

DIRECTIONS

1. Remove the core of the apples and set aside
2. In a bowl combine the rest of the ingredients for the filling
3. Stuff apples with the filling
4. Bake at 400 F until the apple are soft
5. When ready remove from the oven and serve

Serves: **4**

Prep Time: **5** Minutes

Cook Time: **5** Minutes

Total Time: **10** Minutes

INGREDIENTS

- 1-inch ginger-root
- 2 tablespoons lemon juice
- 1 tablespoon honey
- 1 tsp brown sugar

DIRECTIONS

1. Crush the ginger root and pour hot water
2. Add honey, brown sugar and lemon juice
3. Let it chill for 5 minutes and serve

Serves: *8*

Prep Time: *10*   Minutes

Cook Time: *30*   Minutes

Total Time: *40*   Minutes

INGREDIENTS

- 2 cups almond flour
- 1 tsp baking powder
- 1 zucchini
- 1 tablespoon flaxseed
- 1 tablespoon honey
- 1 tsp oregano

DIRECTIONS

1. In a bowl combine water and flaxseed meal
2. Add all dry and wet ingredients, mix well
3. Pour mixture into 8-10 muffin cups
4. Bake for 20-25 minutes at 400 F
5. When ready remove and serve

Serves: *8*

Prep Time: *10*   Minutes

Cook Time: *30*   Minutes

Total Time: *40*   Minutes

INGREDIENTS

- **2 cups rice flour**
- **¼ cup cornmeal**
- **1 tablespoon baking powder**
- **¼ tsp salt**
- **¼ tsp nutmeg**
- **¼ tsp chili powder**
- **¼ cup cocoa powder**
- **1 tablespoon flaxseed meal**
- **¼ cup honey**
- **¼ cup almond milk**
- **¼ cup coconut oil**
- **¼ cup olive oil**

DIRECTIONS

1. In a bowl combine water and flaxseed meal
2. Add all dry and wet ingredients, mix well
3. Pour mixture into 8-10 muffin cups
4. Bake for 20-25 minutes at 400 F
5. When ready remove and serve

Serves: **6**

Prep Time: **15**   Minutes

Cook Time: **35**   Minutes

Total Time: **50**   Minutes

INGREDIENTS

- **1 cup strawberries**
- **1 tablespoon lime juice**
- **1 tablespoon mint**
- **1 tablespoon ginger**
- **1 tsp vanilla powder**
- **1 tsp arrowroot**

TOPPING

- **1 cup coconut flakes**
- **1 tablespoon maple syrup**

DIRECTIONS

1. **In a bowl combine all ingredients for the cobbler and mix well**

2. In another bowl combine all ingredients for the topping

3. Place the cobbler in a baking dish and spread the topping over the cobbler

4. Bake for 30-35 minutes at 375 F

5. When ready remove from the oven and serve

Serves: *8*

Prep Time: *15*   Minutes

Cook Time: *35*   Minutes

Total Time: *50*   Minutes

INGREDIENTS

- 2 tablespoons flaxseed
- ¼ cup water
- 1 cup sweet potato
- 1 cup apple sauce
- ¼ cup ghee
- 1 tablespoon maple syrup
- 1 cup rice flour
- 1 tsp baking powder
- 2 tsp chai mix
- 1 tsp salt

DIRECTIONS

1. In a bowl combine water and flaxseed meal
2. Add all dry and wet ingredients, mix well

3. Pour mixture into 8-10 muffin cups

4. Bake for 20-25 minutes at 400 F

5. When ready remove and serve

Serves: *8-12*

Prep Time: *10*   Minutes

Cook Time: *20*   Minutes

Total Time: *30*   Minutes

INGREDIENTS

- 1 coconut
- cinnamon

DIRECTIONS

1. Cut the coconut into small slices
2. Sprinkle cinnamon over the coconut slices
3. Roast at 375 F for 20-25 minutes
4. When ready remove and serve

Serves: *4*
Prep Time: *10*   Minutes

Cook Time: *30*   Minutes

Total Time: *40*   Minutes

INGREDIENTS

- 1 cup amaranth
- 2 cups water
- 1 tablespoon ghee
- ¼ tsp cumin
- ¼ inch ginger
- ¼ tsp apple cider vinegar
- 1 tsp turmeric
- 1 tablespoon butter
- Handful of raw pumpkin seeds

DIRECTIONS

1. In a pan melt ghee
2. Add ginger, cumin, amaranth and salt
3. Bring to boil, and the rest of the ingredients

4. Cook for 20-25 minutes or until the mixer is thick

5. When ready remove from heat and serve

Serves: *6-8*

Prep Time: *10*   Minutes

Cook Time: *35*   Minutes

Total Time: *45*   Minutes

INGREDIENTS

- 1 cup frozen berries
- 1 tablespoon olive oil
- 1 egg
- 1 cup coconut milk
- ¼ cup cocnut nectar
- 2 tablespoons coconut flour
- ¼ tsp vanilla extract
- ¼ tsp salt

DIRECTIONS

1. Grease a baking dish with olive oil
2. Add the berries in the baking dish and bake for 8-10 minutes at 375 F
3. In a bowl combine the rest of the ingredients

4. Remove the dish from the oven, pour the batter over and place back in the oven

5. Bake for 20-25 minutes, when ready remove and serve

Serves: *8*

Prep Time: *10* Minutes

Cook Time: *60* Minutes

Total Time: *70* Minutes

INGREDIENTS

- 1 pumpkin
- 1 cup rice
- 1 cup pecans
- 1 cup cranberries
- 1 cup chicken stock
- 1 tsp salt
- 1 tablespoon flax seed
- 1 tablespoon coconut oil

DIRECTIONS

1. Scoop out the seeds from the pumpkin and rub with coconut oil

2. In a bowl combine all ingredients for the stuffing

3. Stuff the pumpkin and bake at 375 F for 50-60 minutes or until the pumpkin is soft

4.   When ready remove from the oven and serve

Serves: *6*
Prep Time: *5*   Minutes

Cook Time: *10*   Minutes

Total Time: *15*   Minutes

INGREDIENTS

- 1 apple
- 1 cup almond flour
- ¼ tsp baking powder
- ¼ tsp salt
- 2 eggs
- 1 tablespoon olive oil

DIRECTIONS

1. In a bowl combine all ingredients together
2. In a skillet heat olive oil and pour 1/6 batter
3. Cook for 1-2 minutes per side
4. When ready remove from the skillet and serve

Serves: **8**

Prep Time: **10** Minutes

Cook Time: **50** Minutes

Total Time: **60** Minutes

INGREDIENTS

- 2 sweet potatoes
- 2 tablespoons olive oil
- 1 tsp cumin
- 1 tsp oregano

DIRECTIONS

1. Toss the potatoes with olive oil, cumin and oregano
2. Lay potatoes slices on a parchment paper
3. Bake at 400 F for 40-50 minutes or until golden brown
4. When ready remove from the oven and serve

Serves: *4*
Prep Time: *10*   Minutes

Cook Time: *30*   Minutes

Total Time: *40*   Minutes

INGREDIENTS

- 2 bananas
- 1 tablespoon olive oil
- ¼ tsp baking powder
- ¼ tsp salt
- ½ cup coconut flour
- 1 tablespoon coconut flakes

DIRECTIONS

1. In a bowl combine wet and dry ingredients together and mix well
2. Pour mixture into 8-10 muffin cups
3. Bake for 20-25 minutes at 400 F
4. When ready remove and serve

Serves: **2**
Prep Time: **5**   Minutes

Cook Time: **15**   Minutes

Total Time: **20**   Minutes

INGREDIENTS

- ¼ cup chia seeds
- 1 cup coconut milk
- ¼ tsp vanilla essence
- 1 tsp honey
- 1 handful of berries

DIRECTIONS

1. In a bowl combine chia seeds with warm milk and honey
2. Add the rest of the ingredients and pour into a pot
3. Cook on low heat for 12-15 minutes
4. When ready remove from heat and serve

GRASSFED BEEF & QUINOA CHILI

Serves: *6*

Prep Time: *10* Minutes

Cook Time: *30* Minutes

Total Time: *40* Minutes

INGREDIENTS

- 1 onion
- 2 cloves garlic
- 1 lb. ground grassfed beef
- 1 tsp salt
- 1 tablespoon chili powder
- 1 tablespoon cumin
- 1 can diced tomatoes
- 1 can tomato sauce
- 1 cup water
- 2 cans kidney beans

DIRECTIONS

1. In a pot sauté onion and garlic until soft

2. Add spices, beef and chili powder

3. Stir in tomato sauce, tomatoes, beans and simmer for
    15-20 minutes

4. When thickens remove from heat and serve with
    guacamole

Serves: *4*

Prep Time: *5*   Minutes

Cook Time: *15*   Minutes

Total Time: *20*   Minutes

INGREDIENTS

- 1 cup orzo pasta
- ¼ cup basil leaves
- ¼ cup sun-dried tomatoes
- 1 tablespoon olive oil
- ¼ cup parmesan cheese
- ¼ tsp salt
- ¼ tsp black pepper

DIRECTIONS

1. In a pot bring water to a boil, add orzo and cook for 10 minutes

2. In a blender add basil leaves, sun-dried tomatoes and blend until smooth

3. In a bowl toss together the orzo, and basil mixture with olive oil and parmesan cheese

4. Serve when ready

Serves: **2**

Prep Time: **10**   Minutes

Cook Time: **20**   Minutes

Total Time: **30**   Minutes

INGREDIENTS

- 1 lb. pack chicken pieces
- ¼ tsp chili powder
- 1 garlic clove
- 1 tsp olive oil
- 2 wraps
- 1 avocado
- 1 roasted red pepper

DIRECTIONS

1. In a bowl combine chicken, chili powder, lime juice and garlic
2. In a pan heat oil and fry the chicken mixture
3. Add mixture to each wrap and top with avocado and red pepper

Serves: *4*

Prep Time: *10*   Minutes

Cook Time: *20*   Minutes

Total Time: *30*   Minutes

INGREDIENTS

- 100g penne
- 1 tsp olive oil
- 1 onion
- 1 pepper
- 1 garlic clove
- 1 tsp chili powder
- 1 tsp coriander
- ¼ tsp cumin seeds
- 1 lb. tomatoes
- 1 can sweetcorn
- 1 avocado
- ¼ lime

DIRECTIONS

1. Cook the pasta for 10-15 minutes
2. In a pan heat oil and sautéed onion, garlic and tomatoes
3. Stir in water, corn and simmer for another 12-15 minutes
4. Toss the avocado with lime juice
5. Place the pasta in the pot, add remaining ingredients, cook for another 2-3 minutes
6. When ready remove from heat and serve

Serves: *2*
Prep Time: *10*   Minutes

Cook Time: *15*   Minutes

Total Time: *25*   Minutes

INGREDIENTS

- 2 tuna fillets
- 1 avocado
- 1 tsp mustard powder
- 1 tsp apple cider vinegar
- 6 romaine lettuce leaves
- 8-10 cherry tomatoes

DIRECTIONS

1. In a pan add took and cook for 1-2 minutes per side
2. Combine avocado with vinegar, mustard powder and mix well
3. Spoon avocado mixture into lettuce leaves and top with tomatoes
4. When ready serve with tuna

Serves: *1*

Prep Time: *5*   Minutes

Cook Time: *5*   Minutes

Total Time: *10*   Minutes

INGREDIENTS

- 2 cups cooked chicken breast
- 1 cup mayonnaise
- 1 tsp paprika
- 1 cup celery
- 1 green onion
- ¼ cup green bell pepper
- 1 cup pecans

DIRECTIONS

1. In a bowl mix all ingredients and mix well
2. Serve with dressing

Serves: *1*

Prep Time: *5*   Minutes

Cook Time: *5*   Minutes

Total Time: *10*   Minutes

INGREDIENTS

- 1 egg
- 1 can tuna
- 2 tablespoons mayonnaise
- 2 stalks celery
- Pinch of salt

DIRECTIONS

1. In a bowl mix all ingredients and mix well
2. Serve with dressing

Serves: *1*

Prep Time: *5*   Minutes

Cook Time: *5*   Minutes

Total Time: *10*   Minutes

INGREDIENTS

- ¼ cup apple cider vinegar
- ¼ cup vegetable oil
- ¼ tsp paprika
- ¼ cup almonds
- 1-quart strawberries
- 1 romaine lettuce

DIRECTIONS

1. In a bowl mix all ingredients and mix well
2. Serve with dressing

Serves: *1*

Prep Time: **5**   Minutes

Cook Time: **5**   Minutes

Total Time: ***10***   Minutes

INGREDIENTS

- 4 beets
- 2 tablespoons balsamic vinegar
- 1 tsp maple syrup
- ¼ cup tomatoes
- ¼ cup cucumber

DIRECTIONS

1. In a bowl mix all ingredients and mix well
2. Serve with dressing

Serves: *1*

Prep Time: *5*   Minutes

Cook Time: *5*   Minutes

Total Time: *10*   Minutes

INGREDIENTS

- ½ cabbage
- ¼ red onion
- 1 carrot
- 1 tablespoon cilantro
- ¼ lemon

DIRECTIONS

1. In a bowl mix all ingredients and mix well
2. Serve with dressing

Serves: *1*

Prep Time: **5**   Minutes

Cook Time: **5**   Minutes

Total Time: **10**   Minutes

INGREDIENTS

- 1 package fusilli pasta
- 2 cups tomatoes
- ¼ cup cheese
- ¼ lb. salami
- 1 green bell pepper
- 1 can black olives
- 1 can salad dressing

DIRECTIONS

1. In a bowl mix all ingredients and mix well
2. Serve with dressing

Serves: *1*

Prep Time: *5*   Minutes

Cook Time: *5*   Minutes

Total Time: *10*   Minutes

INGREDIENTS

- 2 cucumber
- 1 cup feta cheese
- 1 cup olive
- ¼ cup red onion
- 1 tablespoon olive oil

DIRECTIONS

1. **In a bowl mix all ingredients and mix well**
2. **Serve with dressing**

Serves: *1*
Prep Time: **5**   Minutes

Cook Time: **5**   Minutes

Total Time: **10**   Minutes

INGREDIENTS

- ¼ cup almonds
- 1 lb. spinach
- 1 cup cranberries
- 1 tablespoon sesame seeds
- ¼ tsp paprika
- ¼ cup apple cider vinegar

DIRECTIONS

1. In a bowl mix all ingredients and mix well
2. Serve with dressing

Serves: *1*

Prep Time: *5* Minutes

Cook Time: *5* Minutes

Total Time: *10* Minutes

INGREDIENTS

- 10 oz. black beans
- 10 oz. corn kernels
- 10 oz. kidney beans
- 1 green bell pepper
- 1 red bell pepper
- 1 red onion
- ¼ cup olive oil
- 1 tablespoon lime juice
- ¼ tsp chili powder

DIRECTIONS

1. In a bowl mix all ingredients and mix well
2. Serve with dressing

Serves: *1*

Prep Time: *5*   Minutes

Cook Time: *5*   Minutes

Total Time: *10*   Minutes

INGREDIENTS

- 2 cups cooked macaroni
- 1 cup mayonnaise
- ¼ cup vinegar
- 1 tsp salt
- 1 onion
- 2 celery stalks
- ½ cup carrot

DIRECTIONS

1. In a bowl mix all ingredients and mix well
2. Serve with dressing

Serves: *1*

Prep Time: **5**   Minutes

Cook Time: **5**   Minutes

Total Time: **10**   Minutes

INGREDIENTS

- 4 eggs
- 1 lb. bacon
- 1 onion
- 1 stalk celery
- 1 cup mayonnaise
- salt

DIRECTIONS

1. **In a bowl mix all ingredients and mix well**
2. **Serve with dressing**

Serves: *1*

Prep Time: **5**   Minutes

Cook Time: **5**   Minutes

Total Time: **10**   Minutes

INGREDIENTS

- 4 eggs
- ¼ lb. bacon
- ½ red onion
- 1 head broccoli
- 1 cup mayonnaise
- salt

DIRECTIONS

1. In a bowl mix all ingredients and mix well
2. Serve with dressing

CUCUMBER SOUP

Serves: **2**

Prep Time: **10**   Minutes

Cook Time: **20**   Minutes

Total Time: **30**   Minutes

INGREDIENTS

- 2 tablespoons olive oil
- 2 cloves garlic
- ¼ cup lemon juice
- ¼ cup parsley
- ¼. cup cilantro
- ¼ cup greens
- 1 cup baby spinach
- 2 cups cucumber
- Salt
- radishes

DIRECTIONS

1. In a blender add all ingredients and blend until smooth
2. Season and refrigerate the soup
3. When ready pour soup into bowl and serve

Serves: *4*
Prep Time: *10*   Minutes

Cook Time: *40*   Minutes

Total Time: *50*   Minutes

INGREDIENTS

- 1 lb. bison
- 1 tablespoon olive oil
- ¼ cabbage
- 2 carrots
- 1 onion
- 2 cloves garlic
- 2 tablespoons aminos
- 4 cups chicken stock

DIRECTIONS

1. In a pot sauté the carrot, onion and cabbage for 2-3 minutes
2. Add bison and cook for 4-5 minutes
3. Add chicken stock, garlic, ginger and coconut aminos
4. Cook for 25-30 minutes

5. When ready from heat garnish with pepper and serve

62

Serves: *4*

Prep Time: *10*   Minutes

Cook Time: *40*   Minutes

Total Time: *50*   Minutes

INGREDIENTS

- 1 tablespoon olive oil
- 1 cup carrot
- 1 cup onion
- 1 cup celery
- 1 chicken breast
- 2 cloves garlic
- 6 cups chicken broth
- ½ cup brown rice
- ¼ cup lemon juice
- 1 tsp black pepper
- ¼ cup parsley

DIRECTIONS

1. In a pot sauté the carrot, onion and celery for 2-3 minutes

2. Add chicken breast and cook for another 4-5 minutes

3. Add rice, lemon juice, pepper and chicken broth

4. Cook for 30-40 minutes on high heat

5. When soup is cooked remove from heat

6. Garnish with parsley and serve

Serves: **2**

Prep Time: **10**   Minutes

Cook Time: **20**   Minutes

Total Time: **30**   Minutes

INGREDIENTS

- 2 tablespoons arame
- 1 cup water
- 2 cups chicken broth
- 1 cup mushrooms
- 2 tablespoons miso paste
- 10 oz. codfish fillet
- 2 cups vegetables
- ¼ cup broccoli sprouts
- 1 tablespoon scallion
- 1 tablespoon olive oil

DIRECTIONS

1. In a bowl soak arame and set aside
2. In a saucepan add broth and bring to a boil

3. Add the cod to the saucepan, vegetables. cover and cook for 5-6 minutes

4. Stir in the miso paste and cook until soup is ready

5. Ladle into bowls top with scallions and serve

Serves: **6**

Prep Time: **20**   Minutes

Cook Time: **35**   Minutes

Total Time: **55**   Minutes

INGREDIENTS

- 2 tablespoons olive oil
- 2 onions
- 2 celery sticks
- 4 garlic cloves
- 4 sprigs of rosemary
- 3 carrots
- 3 cups mushrooms
- 4 cups vegetable broth
- 2 bay leaves

DIRECTIONS

1. In a saucepan sauté garlic, celery, onions until soft
2. Add mushrooms, carrots and sauté for another 4-5 minutes
3. Add bay leaves, broth and simmer for 25-30 minutes

4.   When ready remove from heat and serve

Serves: *4*

Prep Time: *15*   Minutes

Cook Time: *50*   Minutes

Total Time: *65*   Minutes

INGREDIENTS

- 1 chicken
- 2 tablespoons coconut oil
- 2 l water
- 2 tablespoons apple cider vinegar
- 2 onions
- 6 carrots
- 5 celery sticks
- 2 zucchinis
- 1-inch ginger root
- 4 cloves garlic
- 1 bunch parsley

DIRECTIONS

1. Cut chicken into pieces and place in a pot

2. Add water, vinegar, parsley and boil for 50-60 minutes

3. Meanwhile add the rest of the ingredients

4. Simmer for 5-6 hours on low heat

5. When ready remove from heat and serve

Serves: *4*

Prep Time: *10*   Minutes

Cook Time: *50*   Minutes

Total Time: *60*   Minutes

INGREDIENTS

- 8 oz. fennel bulbs
- 10 oz. asparagus
- 1 bunch onions
- 3 cups water
- 1 tsp salt
- 2 tablespoons rice
- 2 leeks
- 2 tablespoons sesame oil
- ¼ cup dill
- ¼ cup mint leaves
- 2 cups vegetable broth
- 2 tablespoons lemon juice

DIRECTIONS

1. In a skillet heat olive oil and sauté onion, dill and mint leaves

2. Slice the vegetables and place them in a pot

3. Add salt, rice, water and simmer for 35-45 minutes

4. Add sautéed ingredients to the soup and simmer for another 4-5 minutes

5. When ready blend the soup and serve

Serves: *2*

Prep Time: *15*   Minutes

Cook Time: *20*   Minutes

Total Time: *35*   Minutes

INGREDIENTS

- 2 cups water
- 1 tablespoon soy sauce
- 2 oz. seaweed
- ¼ cup tofu
- 1-inch ginger
- 1 tsp olive oil
- 2 garlic cloves
- 4 scallions

DIRECTIONS

1. In a soup pot add water, scallion, ginger, garlic and bring to a boil
2. In a skillet heat olive oil and sauté tofu
3. Add sautéed tofu to the soup and the rest of the ingredients

4. Cook until soup is cooked

5. When ready remove from heat garnish with scallions
    and serve

Serves: **8**

Prep Time: **10** Minutes

Cook Time: **30** Minutes

Total Time: **40** Minutes

INGREDIENTS

- 1 lb. beef
- 2 garlic cloves
- 2 cups beef broth
- 2 cups tomatoes
- 1 tsp basil
- ¼ tsp oregano
- 2 cups bow tie pasta
- 2 cups spinach

DIRECTIONS

1. In a pot cook garlic, beef and for 5-6 minutes
2. Stir in tomatoes, broth, pasta and bring to a boil
3. Cook for 8-10 minutes or until pasta is tender
4. Stir in spinach and cook for another 4-5 minutes

5. When ready remove from heat, garnish with basil and
    serve

Serves: *6*
Prep Time: *10*   Minutes

Cook Time: *30*   Minutes

Total Time: *40*   Minutes

INGREDIENTS

- 1 lb. ground beef
- ¼ tsp salt
- ½ tsp garlic powder
- ½ tsp pepper
- 1 tablespoon olive oil
- 1 onion
- 4 cups cabbage
- 2 cups green chilies
- 2 cups water
- 1 can beef broth
- 1 tablespoon cilantro

DIRECTIONS

1. In a saucepan cook beef for 7-8 minutes

2. Add onion, cabbage and sauté for 5-6 minutes

3. Add chilies, broth, water and bring to a boil

4. Stir in cilantro and simmer on low heat for 12-15 minutes

5. When ready remove from heat and serve

Serves: *6*
Prep Time: *10*   Minutes

Cook Time: *30*   Minutes

Total Time: *40*   Minutes

INGREDIENTS

- ¼ lb. bacon strips
- ½ cup onion
- 1 lb. potatoes
- 1 can corn
- 1 can evaporated milk
- ¼ tsp pepper

DIRECTIONS

1. Cook bacon until crispy, when ready remove from heat
2. Add onion and cook until soft
3. Add potatoes, water and bring to a boil
4. Cook for 15-20 minutes
5. Add the rest of the ingredients to the saucepan including bacon and cook until the soup is cooked

6.   When ready remove from heat and serve

Serves: *2*

Prep Time: *10*   Minutes

Cook Time: *20*   Minutes

Total Time: *30*   Minutes

INGREDIENTS

- ¼ cup olive oil
- ½ cup all-purpose flour
- 1 tsp curry powder
- ¼ tsp onion powder
- 1 can tomato juice
- croutons

DIRECTIONS

1. In a saucepan heat olive oil
2. Add, flour, onion powder and curry powder
3. Add tomato juice and cook until soup thickens
4. When ready remove from heat and serve with croutons

GREEN SMOOTHIE

Serves: *1*

Prep Time: *5*   Minutes

Cook Time: *5*   Minutes

Total Time: *10*   Minutes

INGREDIENTS

- 2 celery stalks
- ¼ cup parsley
- ¼ lemon
- ¼ avocado
- 1 cup romaine lettuce
- 1 cup coconut water
- 1 cup ice

DIRECTIONS

1. In a blender place all ingredients and blend until smooth
2. Pour smoothie in a glass and serve

Serves: *1*

Prep Time: *5*   Minutes

Cook Time: *5*   Minutes

Total Time: *10*   Minutes

INGREDIENTS

- ½ cup blueberries
- 1 cup romaine lettuce
- 1 celery stalk
- ¼ tsp cinnamon
- 1 tablespoon almond butter
- 1 cup unsweetened coconut milk

DIRECTIONS

1. In a blender place all ingredients and blend until smooth
2. Pour smoothie in a glass and serve

Serves: *1*

Prep Time: **5**   Minutes

Cook Time: **5**   Minutes

Total Time: **10** Minutes

INGREDIENTS

- 1 cup pineapple
- 1 cup coconut milk
- 2 celery stalks
- 1 tablespoon coconut oil
- 1 cup ice

DIRECTIONS

1. In a blender place all ingredients and blend until smooth
2. Pour smoothie in a glass and serve

Serves: *1*

Prep Time: **5**   Minutes

Cook Time: **5**   Minutes

Total Time: ***10***   Minutes

INGREDIENTS

- 1 cup unsweetened coconut milk
- 2 celery stalks
- 1 tsp cinnamon
- 1 tablespoon almond butter
- ¼ cup coconut flakes

DIRECTIONS

1. In a blender place all ingredients and blend until smooth
2. Pour smoothie in a glass and serve

Serves: *1*

Prep Time: *5*   Minutes

Cook Time: *5*   Minutes

Total Time: *10*   Minutes

INGREDIENTS

- 1 tablespoon tyrosine
- ½ cup kale
- ½ cup watercress
- 1 cup ice
- ½ cup water

DIRECTIONS

1. **In a blender place all ingredients and blend until smooth**
2. **Pour smoothie in a glass and serve**

Serves: *1*

Prep Time: *5*   Minutes

Cook Time: *5*   Minutes

Total Time: *10*   Minutes

INGREDIENTS

- 4 oz. Greek yogurt
- 1 banana
- ¼ cup oats
- ¼ cup pineapple
- ¼ cup unsweetened coconut milk
- 1 cup ice

DIRECTIONS

1. **In a blender place all ingredients and blend until smooth**
2. **Pour smoothie in a glass and serve**

Serves: *1*

Prep Time: *5*   Minutes

Cook Time: *5*   Minutes

Total Time: *10*   Minutes

INGREDIENTS

- 1 cup apple cider
- ¼ Greek yogurt
- ¼ cup oats
- 1 tablespoon pecans
- ¼ tsp cinnamon
- ½ apple

DIRECTIONS

1. **In a blender place all ingredients and blend until smooth**
2. **Pour smoothie in a glass and serve**

Serves: *1*

Prep Time: *5*   Minutes

Cook Time: *5*   Minutes

Total Time: *10* Minutes

INGREDIENTS

- 2 kiwi fruit
- 1 mango
- 400 ml pineapple juice
- 1 banana

DIRECTIONS

1. In a blender place all ingredients and blend until smooth
2. Pour smoothie in a glass and serve